HEAL AND PROTECT YOUR HEART AND NERVOUS SYSTEM.

Easy-to-Apply and Simplified Scientific Based Steps to Maintain and Repair Damaged Heart and Nervous System

Maria L. White

Table of contents

PART 1

OVERVIEW

Nervous System
Whatever you do involves your nervous system. Your nervous system consists of three primary components: your brain, spinal cord, and nerves. You can move, think, and feel better with it. It even controls bodily functions you don't think about, including

digestion. Both the peripheral and central
nerve systems are contained inside it.
The body's nervous system, which consists of
the peripheral and central nervous systems.
Your brain, spinal cord, and nerves are all
part of your nervous system.

Chapter 1

What does the nervous system consist of?

Your body's central nervous system is its command center. It is composed of nerves, spinal cord, and brain. Your nervous system communicates with every other part of your body by transmitting electrical impulses, or messages, from your brain to every other portion. These cues instruct you to do things like breathe, move, speak, and see. Your nervous system monitors both internal and external events and determines how to react to any given circumstance.

Complex functions like memory and cognitive processes are regulated by your nervous system. It is also crucial for the automatic bodily functions including blushing, perspiration, and blinking.

Chapter 2

Operation
The nervous system performs what?

The primary job of your nervous system is to relay instructions to your body from different sections of your body to your brain and vice versa. These communications control your:

•Feelings

•Memories

• Learning

• Thoughts.

Motions (emotional control and equilibrium).

Senses:

 the way your mind processes information from your taste, touch, hearing, and sight.

•wound recovery.

Rest.

respiration and heart rate patterns

reaction to tense circumstances, which
includes perspiration
Breakdown.
physiological processes including aging and
puberty.

Chapter 3

What is the nervous system's mechanism?

Your nervous system sends messages, or signals, throughout your body through neurons, which are nerve cells. These electrical impulses pass through your muscles, glands, organs, skin, and brain. You are able to move your limbs and experience discomfort thanks to the communications. You take in information about your surroundings through your eyes, hearing, tongue, nose, and all of the nerves throughout your body. Nerves then transfer that information to and from your brain.

Neurones come in a variety of forms. Each kind of neuron performs a distinct function:

Your muscles get messages from your motor neurons in the brain and spinal cord. They facilitate your movement. Additionally, they support speech, swallowing, and breathing.

Motor and sensory neurons communicate through interneurons. These neurons affect how you learn, think, and remember things. They also control how you move in reaction to sensory input, such as turning away from a scorching surface.

Anatomy

Which components make up the nervous system?

Two primary components make up the nervous system:

The brain and spinal cord comprise the central nervous system (CNS). Your brain

controls your thoughts, movements, and emotions by interpreting impulses from your nerves.
Your body's peripheral nervous system (PNS) is composed of a network of nerves.

The spinal cord gives birth to branches of nerves. Your arms, legs, fingers, and toes receive information from your brain and spinal cord through this system.
Your peripheral nerve system is divided into two sections:

Your voluntary motions are controlled by your somatic nervous system.
Your actions that you perform unconsciously are controlled by your autonomic nervous system (involuntary movements).

Chapter 4

What is the structure of the nervous system?

The fundamental units of your neurological system are nerve cells, or neurons. Your brain contains 100 billion neurons. Your body's cells are connected throughout.

Consider the neural system in your body as a tree. Like the trunk of a tree, your brain and spinal cord are part of your central nervous system. Your peripheral nervous system, or nerves, are the tree branches. All of your body's parts are reached via the branches that emanate from the truck, which is your spinal cord and brain.

Chapter 5

Situations and Infirmities

Which illnesses or ailments commonly impact the neurological system?

Your neural system might be impacted by a variety of situations. The most popular ones are as follows:

- Dementia.
- Cancer.
- Palsy cerebral.
- Seizures.
- Alzheimer's disease.
- (Meningitis) infection.
- Parkinson's illness.
- Stroke.
- Traumatic brain damage.

Chapter 6

What symptoms or indicators of disorders of the neurological system are typical?

Depending on the disease, signs and symptoms of nervous system disorders might include:

•Changes occur in coordination and movement.
•Loss of memory.
•Sensations such as pain, numbness, or pins and needles.
•Alterations in behavior and mood.
•Thinking and reasoning challenges.

Fits.
Certain diseases require immediate medical attention, such as strokes. Call 911 or your

local emergency services number if you
experience any of the following symptoms:

•Your body's one side experiencing paralysis
or muscle weakness.
•abrupt loss of vision.
•Speech slurred.

Chapter 7

Which tests evaluate your nervous system's health?

Your nervous system's condition may be assessed by a medical professional using one of the following tests:

CAT scan (computerized tomography).
Electrocardiogram, also known as an EKG.
the electroencephalogram (EEG).
The spinal tap, or lumbar puncture.
magnetic resonance imaging scans (MRIs).

Chapter 8

What is the treatment plan for disorders affecting the neurological system?

Your nervous system may be affected by illnesses that a medical professional will identify and treat after reviewing your symptoms. Every ailment requires a different approach. When developing your treatment plan, your healthcare professional will therefore take into account a number of criteria, including your age and general health.

This scheme might consist of:

•taking prescription drugs.
•undergoing surgery.
•taking part in counseling to receive emotional and psychological assistance.

•obtaining supportive care in order to
maintain your comfort.

Chapter 9

Take Care

How can I maintain the health of my nerve system?

By seeing a doctor on a regular basis, you can maintain the health of your neurological system.
1.Preserving health (e.g., by consuming a balanced diet).
2. Avoiding dangerous materials (such as quitting smoking).
3. Wearing safety gear, such as a helmet, when engaging in specific activities or sports.
4. Taking care of any underlying medical issues.

When ought to contact a medical professional?

In the event that you observe any abrupt
changes in your health, such as:

•Weakening of the muscles.
•Either severe headaches or visual
impairment.
•Slurred words.
•Your arms or legs may become numb, tingly,
or lose all feeling.
•Unpredictable muscle movements,
sometimes known as tics or tremors.
•Behavioral or memory changes.
•Inability to move your muscles or with
coordination.

Contact your local emergency services
number or 911 if you or a loved one exhibits
symptoms of a seizure or stroke.

An announcement from Cleveland Clinic

Your body's central nervous system serves as its command center. It supports your ability to move, think, learn, and recall.

Conclusion

Your entire system of muscles, glands, and organs is connected by this enormous network of nerves. To continue operating, it requires maintenance. Unexpected things like an infection, accident, or underlying illness can occasionally have an impact on your neurological system. A medical professional can help you maintain your health so that your nervous system has everything it needs to perform as intended.

PART 2

THE HEART

The heart is a muscular pump that pumps blood throughout the body to all of the tissues. This is an essential function because cells cannot function properly and will eventually die if there is not a constant flow of new blood.

Preventing heart disease and keeping the heart healthy are crucial because they can hinder the heart from working properly.

Chapter 10

HEART DISEASE, TREATMENT AND PREVENTION

HEART ATTACK

A myocardial infarction, often known as a heart attack, is a sudden stoppage of blood flow to a portion of the heart. This usually results from an obstruction that stops blood flow normally, but supply and demand imbalances can also cause it.
The cardiac muscle in that area may start to die if the blood flow does not return to normal.

HEART FAILURE

A condition known as heart failure, or congestive heart failure, occurs when the heart is unable to adequately pump blood throughout the body. This could be the result of the heart not pumping blood efficiently or not filling with enough blood. It does not refer to the stopping of the heart, despite the name.

Research indicates that 6.2 million adults in the United States suffer from heart failure, and that about 805,000 Americans suffer from heart attacks annually. These are two fairly common illnesses.

Causes of Heart Attack:

Heart attacks can be caused by a wide range of factors. One common cause of heart attacks is coronary artery disease, which occurs when plaque builds up in the coronary arteries, narrowing or blocking the arteries' ability to carry oxygen-rich blood to the heart. Another common cause of heart attacks is coronary artery spasm, which occurs when a coronary artery's walls severely tighten or spasm, cutting off blood flow through the artery.

Causes of heart failure

Heart failure can also be caused by a variety of circumstances. It usually results from an injury or infection that damages the heart, or from other medical disorders that make the heart to work too hard.

Both the left and right sides of the heart may be impacted by heart failure. While the right side gathers blood with low oxygen content and pumps it to the lungs to obtain oxygen, the left side circulates blood rich in oxygen throughout the body.

Heart failure is more likely to impact the left side of the body and the heart's ability to

pump blood efficiently. Left-sided heart
failure comes in two flavors: reduced ejection
fraction and preserved ejection fraction,
according to a reliable source.

Systolic heart failure, commonly referred to
as reduced ejection fraction, is the inability of
the heart to contract efficiently. This could be
because of:
coronary heart disease
genetic cardiomyopathy
defective valves in the heart
erratic pulse
developed cardiac conditions
Methamphetamine, cocaine, alcohol, or other
poisons
The condition known as preserved ejection
fraction, or diastolic heart failure, occurs
when the heart is unable to contract
completely. As a result, it cannot pump as
much blood to the body as it would like to.
This could be because of:

•hypertension,
•obesity, and diabetes.
The heart cannot pump enough blood to the lungs to take up adequate oxygen when there is right-sided heart failure. It commonly happens as a result of left-sided cardiac failure. Blood clots in the blood arteries that convey blood from the heart to the lungs are the cause of this increase in pressure.

Signs of a heart attack

Not all heart attacks have obvious symptoms when they first occur. These could be referred to by doctors as quiet heart attacks. A heart attack's symptoms can differ from person to person. Individuals with a history of heart attacks may experience distinct symptoms. Generally speaking, the most prevalent symptoms are:

upper-body discomfort, including pain in the arms, shoulders, neck, jaw, or stomach, as well as shortness of breath in the chest Additional signs and symptoms could be:

•perspiring exhaustion
•vomiting and nausea
•unexpected dizziness or •lightheadedness

Signs of heart failure

The nature and intensity of the ailment determine the heart failure symptoms. Breathlessness is a typical sign of heart failure, both left and right sided. Usually, as the heart weakens, the symptoms worsen.

Among the signs of left-sided heart failure are:

•overall lassitude
•breathing difficulties

•tiredness
•difficulty focusing
•bluish finger and lip hue due to exhaustion
from coughing
•having trouble falling asleep

The following are possible signs of
right-sided heart failure:

•edema
•weight gain
•nausea
•appetite decline
•stomach ache
•Having frequent urination

Identification

A doctor will probably identify a heart attack
based on the patient's signs, symptoms, and
medical history because of the urgency of a

possible heart attack. They are also capable of doing diagnostic exams.

An electrocardiogram (EKG), blood tests, stress tests, or coronary angiography may be necessary for this.

Analogously, a physician can identify heart failure based on a patient's medical history, physical examination, and diagnostic tests.

Typically, an echocardiography and blood tests from Trusted Source are part of this testing. A doctor may then prescribe more testing, such as an MRI, CT scan, EKG, or stress tests, if these tests yield no clear results.

Therapy for heart attacks

Prompt heart attack treatment can help avoid or lessen serious damage to the heart muscle.

Prior to a heart attack being diagnosed, a patient may receive treatment for:

beta-blockers, aspirin, nitroglycerin, and oxygen therapy
A physician will attempt to reduce or remove the blockage in order to restore blood flow after making a diagnosis. Medication, coronary angioplasty, and intervention might be part of this.

A balloon is used during a medical treatment called coronary angioplasty to widen the artery and start blood flow again. To maintain the artery open, a physician may also implant a stent, which is a tiny mesh tube.

Additionally, a physician might recommend medication to lessen blood pressure, lessen clotting, and lessen cardiac strain.

Therapy for heart failure

While there is no known cure for heart failure, there are therapies that can prolong a patient's life while reducing symptoms. Depending on the type of heart failure a person has, treatment options will vary; nevertheless, medications, lifestyle modifications, and occasionally surgery are the usual options.

When to consult a physician
Heart attacks and heart failure are dangerous illnesses. They can be deadly if left untreated. A healthcare provider should be consulted right away by anyone exhibiting signs of a heart attack or heart failure. The likelihood of recovery can significantly change if treatment is received quickly.

Although they belong to the same category as heart disease, heart attacks and heart failure are distinct disorders.

Heart failure occurs when the heart is unable to pump blood throughout the body effectively, whereas heart attacks occur when the heart does not receive enough blood to function.

Heart attacks and heart failure are distinct illnesses, despite the fact that they both impact the heart's capacity to circulate blood throughout the body.

A healthy lifestyle that includes a diversified diet, frequent exercise, and little stress can help people lower their risk of developing heart disease, even though the two disorders have different origins.

AROTID PARTS

As plaque accumulates inside the carotid arteries, carotid artery disease develops. Blood rich in oxygen is delivered to the brain through these arteries.

There are two big carotid arteries in the neck, one on each side. Before reaching the brain, each of these arteries divides into an internal and external carotid artery.

A mixture of fat, calcium, cholesterol, and other materials makes up plaque. Atherosclerosis is the term for the process by which plaque accumulates in these arteries over time.

Blood flow is impeded and made more difficult by plaque accumulation in the arteries.

A major risk is posed by a constricted artery since it may restrict or obstruct blood flow to the brain, potentially leading to a stroke.
Symptoms and indicators
A doctor may listen for a little "whooshing" sound in the neck in order to identify a bruit.

A large number of individuals with carotid artery disease initially show no symptoms.

As the disease worsens, carotid artery disease typically begins to show symptoms.

Serious symptoms and indicators that indicate a blockage or severe constriction of the artery include:

Bruit

A bruit is a noise that certain patients with carotid artery disease have in their arteries. A stethoscope will be placed on the neck close to the carotid arteries by the doctor during a physical examination, and they will listen for a faint "whooshing" sound.

Abrasions may indicate that atherosclerosis has decreased the person's ability to pump blood through the artery.

Brief Ischemia Attack

It's possible for some people to have a transient ischemic attack (TIA) before they notice any signs of carotid artery damage.

Though not as severe, a TIA is extremely comparable to a stroke. But prompt medical intervention is still necessary.

The following are signs of a TIA and a stroke:

•a terrible headache that appeared out of
nowhere
•lightheadedness
•imbalance loss
•speech issues, including difficulty seeing out
of one or both eyes, •paralysis or numbness
in the face or limbs, usually on one side of
the body, and immobility of one or more
limbs
Anyone exhibiting these signs should get
medical help right away.

When someone has a transient internal attack
(TIA), the symptoms usually fade away in
the first 24 hours.

Stroke

The symptoms of a stroke are similar to those
of a TIA, but they can have more serious
consequences. Because of the oxygen that is
lost during a stroke, brain damage may be
irreversible.

A stroke can result in long-term incapacity, speech difficulties, or irreversible vision abnormalities. A stroke can sometimes result in death or disability.

Anyone experiencing symptoms of a stroke or transient ischemic attack should get emergency medical attention right once.

Reasons and dangerous elements

The underlying cause of carotid artery disease is plaque accumulation. Even while the elements of plaque are present in blood, they are more prone to congregate in the minuscule areas of arterial injury.
In addition to the long-term impacts of diet and lifestyle choices, hereditary factors also contribute to this harm.
The following are significant risk factors that contribute to artery damage and plaque buildup:

•consuming unhealthy food •smoking
•excessive blood pressure •cholesterol
•diabetes or resistance to insulin
•metabolic syndrome
•lack of exercise
•excess weight
•elderly age-related stress and sleep apnea
An elevated risk of artery disease may also
exist in those with a family history of any
kind of atherosclerosis.

Identification

Early detection of carotid artery disease is
crucial in order to avoid potentially fatal
consequences like stroke.

A physician will inquire about the patient's
past medical conditions and way of living. A
physical examination or other blood tests
may be ordered by the doctor if they suspect

that the patient may be at risk for carotid artery disease.

Examining for bruits is a component of physical examinations. Doctors will request more testing if they listen to the arteries and detect a bruit.

Imaging examinations

To look for narrowing and observe inside the carotid arteries, doctors typically employ one or more imaging studies. Imaging examinations consist of:

Sonography

Sound waves are used in a carotid ultrasonography to provide images of the artery interiors.

As the most popular type of imaging test for carotid artery disease, it may typically help identify any arterial narrowing.

Angiography

A specialized dye is used in an angiography
to enhance the visibility of the arteries in the
image.

Following the injection of the dye, medical
professionals will utilize MRIs, CT scans, or
X-rays to create images of the arteries as the
dye flows through them.
Using this test, physicians can see if there are
any arterial blockages or narrowing.

Handling

In order to prevent consequences that could
be fatal and to stop the condition from getting
worse, treatment for carotid artery disease is
essential.

Dietary and lifestyle modifications are part of the treatment. A person could occasionally need to take medicine or have surgery.

Modification to diet and lifestyle.

A key component of any carotid artery disease treatment program is dietary and lifestyle modifications. A doctor may recommend:
•partaking in a "heart-healthy diet."
•maintaining or gaining weight controlling eleminate diseases, such as diabetes or heart issues
•continuing to be physically active
•quitting smoking, if relevant

Chapter 11

General Guidelines for Diets

A general heart-healthy diet involves limiting the intake of the following foods, according to the National Heart, Lung, and Blood Institute (NHLBI):

•salt
•saturated fats
•trans fatty acids
•more sugars
•whiskey
On a balanced, heart-healthy diet full of items like these, the person should instead concentrate on

•fruits,
•veggies, and entire grains
•low-fat dairy goods
•chicken
•fish

•eggs
•lean meats
•beans
•seeds and nuts

Medications

To aid in the management of carotid artery disease, doctors may also advise medication.

Drugs that prevent blood clotting, like aspirin or clopidogrel, are frequently prescribed.

Depending on the underlying risk factors of an individual, doctors may prescribe extra medications, such as blood pressure or cholesterol control ones.

Medical treatments

One or more medical operations may be necessary to lower the risk for people who exhibit symptoms of carotid artery disease or who are at risk for serious complications.

Among the possible steps are:

stenting and angioplasty
If the patient has severe constriction from
plaque, angioplasty and stenting can help
expand the carotid arteries and enhance blood
flow to the brain.

A thin tube with a small deflated balloon on
its end is inserted into the restricted artery by
medical professionals during an angioplasty
treatment. Once the tube is positioned, the
balloon is inflated to force the plaque against
the arterial wall and aid in the restoration of
blood flow through the artery.
Doctors can insert a stent, or small mesh
tube, in the affected location once the artery
has been widened.

The stent is intended to prevent the artery from narrowing in that particular location by providing internal support and strengthening.

Endoscopic surgery

Endarterectomy is less common and might not be appropriate for all patients. For more severe constriction or obstructions, doctors could advise it.

According to the NHLBI, physicians often only suggest endarterectomy when a patient has at least 50% blockage in their arteries.

The treatment involves the surgeon making an incision in the neck to access the constricted artery.

Once the obstruction has been located, an artery will be cut, and the inner lining will be removed. By doing this, the obstruction's cause is removed, aiding in the restoration of blood flow.

Coronary versus carotid artery disease
Despite sharing a common cause, carotid artery disease and coronary artery disease are distinct conditions. Plaque accumulation in the arteries is the cause of both disorders. They therefore share comparable risk factors.

That being said, coronary artery disease is an accumulation of plaque in the arteries that supply the heart, whereas carotid artery disease is an accumulation of plaque in the arteries that supply the brain.

Chapter 12
Prospects

Giving someone the greatest chance possible requires both receiving therapy and changing one's lifestyle.

Patients with carotid artery disease can help stop the condition from growing worse by adhering to their doctor's treatment plan and changing their lifestyle for the better.

There is no complete treatment for carotid artery disease, not even one that works well. Treatment, however, can lower the chance of important occurrences like stroke.

In brief

The brain's arteries thin or get blocked as a result of carotid artery disease.

The risk of plaque accumulation and carotid artery disease is increased by a number of medical disorders and unhealthy lifestyle choices.

Making dietary and lifestyle modifications to lessen plaque accumulation in the arteries and lower the chance of major consequences, like stroke, is an integral part of successful treatment.

Anyone experiencing weakness or slurred speech—signs indicative of a stroke—should get emergency medical assistance.

A sedentary lifestyle may raise the risk of cardiovascular death.

Individuals who do not engage in leisure-time physical activity may be more likely to die from cardiovascular disease (CVD), with two specific categories being at risk:

Combining medications for chest pain and erectile dysfunction may be harmful to the heart.
Combining certain medications for chest discomfort with erectile dysfunction therapies like Viagra, Levitra, or Cialis can raise your risk of cardiovascular disease.

How the health consequences of sitting can be mitigated by exercising for an additional 15 to 30 minutes each day
Researchers have found that even a small amount of regular exercise—just 15 to 30 minutes a day—can help those who spend

their entire workday sitting down and reduce
their risk of heart disease.